The Ultimate Gastric Bypass Cookbook

Gastric Bypass for Dummies

Over 25 Gastric Bypass Recipes You Can't Resist

BY

Rachael Rayner

License Notes

Table of Contents

Introduction

Gastric bypass surgery is a form of weight loss surgery that many people tend to get every year, especially those that are extremely overweight. However, it is not the first surgery of its kind. The truth is there are many different types of weight loss surgery out there that can help to reduce one's weight such as using a gastric band to decrease the size of one's stomach or by removing part of the stomach entirely.

Regardless of what type of weight loss surgery you have had, most of the time you are going to have to change your diet to accommodate these recent changes. No longer are you able to eat as much food as you want and instead have to be very careful of the foods you eat and consider some of the ingredients that you will have to use. You want to make sure that you do not eat foods that are overly fatty or that are so heavy that they can end up damaging your gastric band.

If you have recently had gastric bypass surgery or any other weight loss surgery, then this is the perfect book for you. Inside of this book you will discover over 25 gastric bypass friendly recipes as well as a few helpful tips to ensure that you make the most out of your new chance at losing weight thanks to your weight loss surgery.

So, without further ado, let's get right into it!

Understanding Gastric Bypass Surgery and the Different Types of Weight Loss Surgery Available

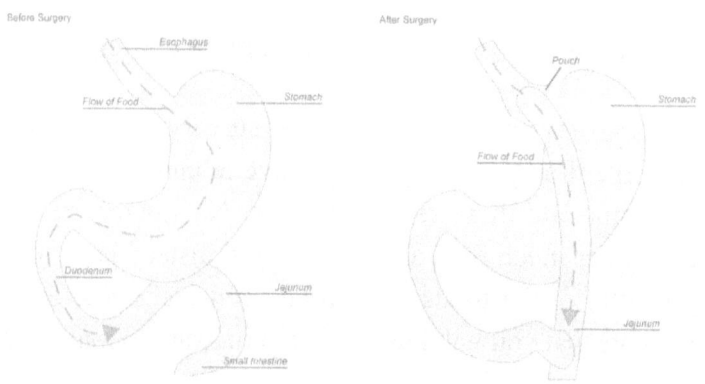

If you are looking into weight loss surgery, then most likely you have already looked into and tried all kinds of dietary and exercise regimens over the past couple of years, but have failed to control your weight. Or even if you have had success in the past you have found that has been short-lived. If you are a person that belongs to the clinically obese category, this means that you may have a chronic disease. The truth of the matter is that if you fit into this category, non-surgical treatment will not work for you and you will have to give some serious thought to potentially having a surgical procedure done on you.

How to Qualify for Gastric Bypass Surgery

In order to qualify for gastric bypass surgery, you need your body mass index to read 40 or more on the scale. Any less than this will not qualify you to have gastric bypass surgery. This number is an indication of how much extra fat you have accumulated within your body. The way that this number is calculated is by aligning your height and your weight to see exactly how much fat is in your body at this particular moment.

If you are a person whose body mass index is less than 18.5, you are within normal weight. However, if you are overweight the reading will show up between 18.5 and 24.9. Anything beyond this number is considered to be obese and is one of the qualifications in order to have gastric bypass surgery.

Also in order to have gastric bypass surgery, your doctor may let you know whether or not a medical condition you are suffering from can be benefited through this type of weight loss such as asthma, sleep apnea, cardiovascular issues, arthritis, gastric reflux, diabetes or even high cholesterol.

Types of Weight Loss Surgeries

You need to keep in mind that gastric bypass is not the only weight loss surgery that you can have. It is only one of many different surgeries that you can have to help you lose weight and begin to become healthier in the long run. In this section you will learn about the various different types of weight-loss surgeries that are available to you so you can choose the surgery that best works for you.

Sleeve Gastrectomy

This type of surgery is a very restrictive surgery. It works by a surgeon making a very small incision in your stomach, cutting out a small piece of your stomach and removing it completely from your body. The portion that is left behind however is given the shape of a tube. This will help to ensure that you cannot consume too much food and it will also reduce the production of an appetite regulating hormone known as ghrelin.

Laparoscopic Banding

This type of restrictive procedure involves placing a band with an inflatable balloon around the upper part of your stomach. This balloon works similar to a pouch and allows food to be lowered into your stomach very slowly. You'll also be able to inflate the balloon via a port that is under the skin of your abdomen.

Duodenal Switch

This type of surgery begins by removing a large portion of your stomach. With the contents left behind your stomach will be responsible for sending any food that you consume through the small intestine as well as to the duodenum. You will then be able to have your duodenum connected to the last part of your small intestine directly which helps to ensure that you decrease the amount of food you are consuming on a daily basis.

Roux-en-Y Gastric Bypass

This type of surgery comprises of creating a very small pouch that sits on top of your stomach. All of the food that you will consume will filter to this spot only and never go anywhere else. What this means is that your digestive juices will still be made within your stomach region and the food that you consume instead will be sent to the small intestine directly.

Tips for Recovering After Your Weight Loss Surgery

Once you have had your weight loss surgery, there are many things that you are going to have to take into consideration as well as be aware of any changes that you are going to have to make. In this section and want to give you a few helpful tips to help you recover from your weight loss surgery as well as make the most of it in the years to come.

1. Always Listen to Your Doctor

The worst thing that you can go through when having this type of surgery is having it and then not losing as much weight as you expected you would lose. This is why it is incredibly important to follow the specific instructions given to you by your doctor so that you can lose as much weight as possible.

With that said you also want to make sure that you never avoid any checkups that you have with your doctor as you can learn more about what is going on within your body as well as your doctor giving you a few more instructions to help increase the amount of weight that you lose. This will help to ensure that you are staying on the right track.

2. Work Only When You Are Ready to Work

If after a couple days after your surgery you are still feeling physically uncomfortable, do not worry about returning to work immediately. You want to take your time with returning to work and with getting back into the regular swing of things. You need to keep in mind that on average it takes about 2 to 3 weeks to be fully healed so don't be afraid to take things slowly at first.

3. Make Sure to get Plenty of Exercise

Once you have fully healed up you want to get into the habit of participating in regular exercise. This will allow your body to strengthen up and deal with the number of calories that you are losing in the process. You don't have to worry about complicated exercise routines. Simple walking on a daily basis will do just fine.

4. Receive Plenty of Support

As with any patient that goes through any type of weight loss surgery, you will need the full support of your family and friends going through it. Never feel bad about asking for help or asking for those close to you to stick around. These people will help you along your journey to weight loss.

5. Make Sure to Take All of Your Medication When You Need To

Another thing that you want to make sure that you are constantly doing is taking your medication each and every time you need to take them. Before stopping any of your medications you want to make sure that you tell your doctor beforehand to ensure that it is not that will affect the results of your weight loss surgery in the first place.

With that said you also want to make sure that you include multivitamins into your daily prescriptions as well. This will help you ensure that you are getting all the nutrition you need even though you are decreasing the amount of food that you are consuming on a daily basis.

6. Don't Drink Alcohol

Last we want to make sure that you avoid drinking any alcohol after your surgery. If you drink alcohol after your surgery you can dramatically affect your recovery time as well as affect how much weight you lose in the process.

7. Keep Track of All of the Calories

Another thing that you want to keep in mind is that with this weight loss surgery you will not be consuming as many calories as you initially would. You want to make sure that you are only consuming at least a minimum of 600 to 800 calories per day or else your surgery will not be successful. Also make sure that you can talk with your doctor to make sure that you are consuming the right number of calories per day to ensure a healthy and successful weight loss.

Healthy Gastric Bypass Recipes

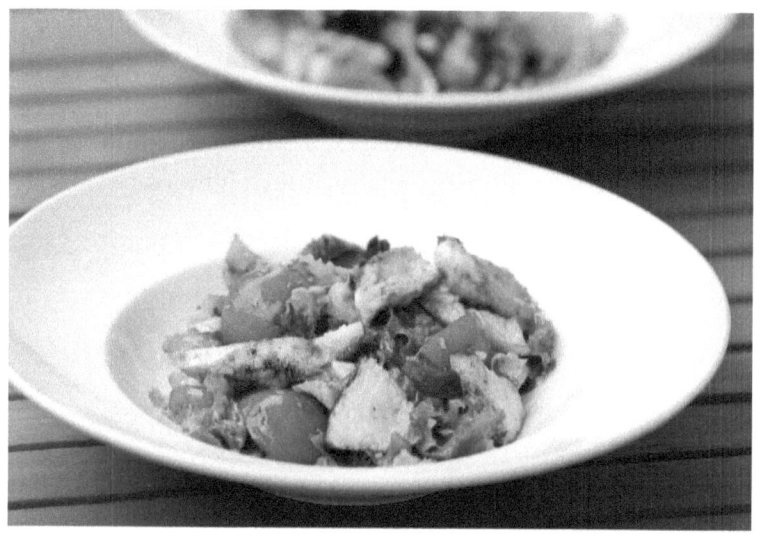

Simple Chocolate Shake

During the liquid phase, you want to make sure you take it easy with the amount of food you consume. This is one liquid phase friendly drink that I know you are going to love it. It is rich in decadent flavor; you won't be able to resist this shake.

Makes: 1 Serving

Total Prep Time: 3 Minutes

Ingredients:

- 1 tsp. of Chocolate, Flavoring
- 1 Scoop of Ice Cream, Vanilla and Optional
- 1 tsp. of Sweetener
- 1 Scoop Protein Powder, Chocolate Variety
- 6 Ounces of Milk, Whole

Directions:

1. Combine all of your ingredients together in a blender.

2. Cover and blend on the highest setting until smooth in consistency.

3. Remove and pour into a chilled glass. Serve right away.

Classic Eggnog

Here is another healthy liquid phase beverage you are going to love especially during the Christmas holidays. It is a classic holiday drink that the entire family can enjoy with you.

Makes: 1 Serving

Total Prep Time: 5 Minutes

Ingredients:

- 5 Cups of Soymilk, Vanilla Flavored and Light
- 6 Packets of Splenda
- 1 Package of Pudding, Instant Variety, Fat Free and Sugar Free
- 1 tsp. of Rum Extract
- ½ tsp. of Nutmeg, Ground

Directions:

1. First use a blender and add all of your ingredients into it.

2. Cover and blend on the highest setting until thoroughly mixed.

3. Place into your fridge to chill for the next couple of hours or until you are ready to serve.

Traditional Tiramisu Coffee

If you are a huge fan of coffee recipes, then this is certainly the recipe for you. It is sweet to taste and packed full of caffeine, making it the perfect early morning drink to enjoy.

Makes: 1 Serving

Total Prep Time: 5 Minutes

Ingredients:

- 4 Ounces of Chocolate Chips, Semisweet Variety
- ½ Cup of Sugar, Powdered
- 16 Ounces of Coffee, Freshly Brewed
- 1 tsp. of Almond Extract
- 4 to 5 Ounces of Liqueur, Coffee Variety
- 8 Ounces of Whipping Cream, Heavy Variety
- 1 Tbsp. of Chocolate, Freshly Grated

Directions:

1. The first thing that you will want to do is melt your chocolate chips in a double boiler with ½ a cup of your coffee.

2. Once melted remove from heat and allow to stand until creamy in consistency.

3. Next mix together your sugar, almond extract and cream in a medium sized bowl. Using an electric mixer and beat at the highest setting until peaks begin to form.

4. Divide up your chocolate mixture amount 4 coffee cups. Add in your remaining coffee and liqueur.

5. Top off with your whipped cream.

6. Garnish with your grated chocolate prior to serving.

Watermelon Sangria

Looking for a tasty alcoholic beverage? Then this is the perfect drink for you to make. Light and hearty, I know you will want to make this drink whenever you are craving one.

Makes: 1 Serving

Total Prep Time: 2 Hours

Ingredients:

- 3 Pounds of Watermelon, Seedless Variety, Peeled, Cubed and Cut into Wedges
- 6 Ounces of Vodka
- Some Ice, Crushed
- 1 Bottle of White Wine, Dry Variety

Directions:

1. Place your watermelon cubes into a blend and blend on the highest setting until thoroughly pureed.

2. Then pour through a find mesh strainer and right into a chilled pitcher.

3. Add in your wine, vodka and ice.

4. Stir until thoroughly mixed and place into your fridge to chill for the next 2 hours.

5. After this time serve whenever you are ready. Enjoy.

Curry Style Vegetable Dip

Here is a great tasting dip that you can serve up when you first enter the mushy phase of eating on your diet. It is easy on your stomach and is packed full of delicious taste that you won't be able to resist.

Makes: 2 Servings

Total Prep Time: 1 Hour

Ingredients:

- 1 Cup of Sour Cream, Reduced in Fat
- 2 Tbsp. of Yellow Mustard, Fully Prepared
- ½ Cup of Mayonnaise, Your Favorite Kind
- 1 tsp. of Curry, Powdered Variety
- 1 Tbsp. of Lemon Juice, Fresh
- ½ tsp. of Paprika
- 2 Tbsp. of Parsley, Roughly Chopped
- ½ tsp. of Tarragon
- 2 Tbsp. of White Onion, Freshly Grated
- Dash of Salt and Pepper, For Taste
- 1 Tbsp. of Chives, Minced

Directions:

1. Use a medium sized bowl and blend together your fresh lemon juice, mayo, sour cream until thoroughly mixed.

2. Then add in your chives, onion, parsley, powdered curry, paprika, tarragon and dash of salt and pepper.

3. Cover and chill for at least 1 hour prior to serving.

Classic Hummus

If you are a fan of traditional hummus, then this is one dip dish you are going to want to enjoy as frequently as possible. Serve this by itself or with something light to make a tasty treat you can enjoy whenever you wish.

Makes: 2 Servings

Total Prep Time: 15 Minutes

Ingredients:

- 1, 16 Ounce Can of Chickpeas, Drained Well
- 2 Cloves of Garlic, Crushed
- ½ tsp. of Salt, For Taste
- 2 Lemons, Fresh and Juice Only
- 2 Tbsp. of Olive Oil, Extra Virgin Variety
- 4 Tbsp. of Tahini

Directions:

1. First combine your fresh lemon juice, canned chickpeas, crushed garlic and dash of salt in a blender and blend on the highest setting for the next minute.

2. Slowly drizzle in your olive oil and continue blending until smooth in consistency.

3. Feel free to add more water if needed.

4. Pour into a serving bowl and create a well in the center. Add your remaining olive oil along with your parsley into the center.

5. Serve whenever you are ready with the food of your choice.

Tasty Bacon Wrapped Jalapeno Poppers

Here is a tasty solid phase recipe that you won't be able to resist. It does have a bit of a spicy taste to it, so it is perfect for those who like their food to contain a little heat.

Makes: 2 Servings

Total Prep Time: 40 Minutes

Ingredients:

- 12 Jalapeno Peppers, Large in Size and Seeded
- 3 Onions, Green in Color and Finely Minced
- 4 Ounces of Cream Cheese, Reduced in Fat and Room Temperature
- 12 Slices of Bacon, Thick Cut
- ½ Cup of Cheddar Cheese, Finely Shredded and Reduced in Fat

Directions:

1. The first thing that you will want to do is cut each jalapeno pepper lengthwise and scoop out both the seeds and membranes.

2. Then use a small sized bowl and mix together your room temperature cream cheese, green onions and cheddar cheese until smooth in consistency.

3. Spoon in some of your cheese filling between each jalapeno pepper. Top off with the halves of your jalapeno peppers.

4. Then wrap a slice of bacon around each pepper. Secure each slice with a toothpick. Place onto a generously greased baking sheet.

5. Preheat your oven to 400 degrees. Once it is hot enough add in your peppers and cook for the next 25 to 30 minutes or until your jalapenos are soft to the touch and your bacon is brown in color.

6. Remove and serve while piping hot. Enjoy.

Chocolate and Soy Dessert

Here is a gastric bypass friendly meal that anybody with a strong sweet tooth will enjoy. It is easy to make and extremely light. I know you won't regret enjoying this dish.

Makes: 2 Servings

Total Prep Time: 35 Minutes

Ingredients:

- 1 Envelope of Gelatin, Unflavored Variety
- ¼ Cup of Water, Hot
- 1 Package of Instant Pudding, Fudge Flavored, Sugar and Fat Free Variety
- 1 Cup of Milk, Cold and Skim Variety
- 16 Ounces of Vanilla, Pure
- 1 Tbsp. of Cocoa, Powdered Variety
- ¼ tsp. of Peppermint Extract, Optional

Directions:

1. Using a small sized bowl, mix together your water and gelatin until thoroughly mixed. Set aside to sit until firm to the touch.

2. Then use another medium sized bowl and mix together your pudding mix and milk until evenly combined.

3. Next dice up your tofu into small sized cubes. Add to your budding mixture and whisk thoroughly to break it up.

4. Add in your vanilla, powdered coca and peppermint. Stir to thoroughly combine.

5. Spoon your tofu and pudding mixture into a food processor. Blend on the highest setting until smooth in consistency. Add this mixture to your gelatin and blend thoroughly until combined.

6. Pour this mixture into a large sized glass dish. Cover with some plastic wrap and place into your fridge to chill for the next 30 minutes.

7. After this time remove from your fridge and serve while cold.

Healthy Tuna and Apple Sandwiches

If you are looking for an easy and delicious sandwich recipe to enjoy, then this is the dish for you. Easy to make and packed full of nutritious ingredients, this is one dish I know you are going to love it.

Makes: 3 Servings

Total Prep Time: 10 Minutes

Ingredients:

- 1, 6.5 Ounce Can of Tuna, packed in Water and Drained
- 1 Apple, Fresh, Peeled, Cored and Diced
- ¼ Cup of Yogurt, Low in Fat and Vanilla Flavored
- 1 tsp. of Mustard
- ½ tsp. of Honey, Raw
- 6 Slices of Bread, Whole Wheat Variety
- 3 Leaves of Lettuce, Fresh

Directions:

1. The first thing that you will want to do is wash and peel your apple. Dice into small sized pieces. Then drain your can of tuna.

2. Add your tuna, diced apples, raw honey, vanilla yogurt and mustard in a medium sized bowl. Stir well to combine.

3. Spread this mixture onto three of your slices of your bread. Top off with your lettuce leaves and remaining bread slices. Serve right away and enjoy.

Healthy Baked Chicken and Vegetables

This is the perfect dish for you to make if you are looking for a perfect and filling dinner dish that will leave you feeling full and satisfied. Packed full of protein and wholesome veggies, this is a healthy lunch and dinner dish that you can serve whenever you wish.

Makes: 6 Servings

Total Prep Time: 1 Hour

Ingredients:

- 4 Potatoes, Russet Variety and Thinly Sliced
- 6 Carrots, Fresh and Thinly Sliced
- 1 Onion, Large in Size and Cut into Quarters
- 1 Chicken, Raw, Skin Removed and Cut into Small Sized Pieces
- ½ Cup of Water, Warm
- 1 tsp. of Thyme, Fresh
- ¼ tsp. of Pepper, For Taste

Directions:

1. The first thing that you will want to do is preheat your oven to 400 degrees.

2. While your oven is heating up add your potatoes, onions and sliced carrots into a large sized roasting pan.

3. Place your chicken on top of your vegetables.

4. Then mix together your dash of pepper, fresh thyme and water together until evenly mixed. Pour this mixture over your chicken and vegetables.

5. Place your dish into your oven and bake for the next hour until your chicken is brown in color and your vegetables are tender to the touch.

6. During the baking process spoon your juices over your chicken at least once or twice.

7. After this time remove from oven and allow to cool slightly before serving. Enjoy.

Classic Asian Lettuce Wraps

If you are looking for something a little more unique and filled with an exotic flavor, then this is the perfect dish for you to make. It is so delicious, I know you are going to want to make it over and over again.

Makes: 4 Servings

Total Prep Time: 25 Minutes

Ingredients:

- 1, 8 Ounce Can of Bamboo Shoots, Drained and Minced
- 1, 8 Ounce Can of Chestnuts, Water Variety, Drained and Minced
- 3 Tbsp. of Cooking Wine, Sherry Variety
- 2 Tbsp. of Hoisin Sauce
- 1 Tbsp. of Peanut Butter, Unsalted Variety
- 2 tsp. of Soy Sauce, Low in Sodium
- 2 tsp. of Hot Sauce, Your Favorite Kind
- 2 Packs of Splenda
- 1 Tbsp. of Garlic, Minced
- 1 Cup of Onion, Minced
- ½ Pound of Chicken Breast, Ground and Lean Variety
- 1 tsp. of Ginger, Minced
- ¼ tsp. of Salt, For Taste
- 1 tsp. of Sesame Oil, Toasted Variety

- 8 Lettuce Leaves, Buttered Variety and Small in Size
- 1 Green Onions, Whole and Finely Chopped
- 1 Cucumber, Seeded and Thinly Sliced

Directions:

1. Use a medium sized bowl and combine your bamboo shoots, sherry wine, hoisin sauce, smooth peanut butter, soy sauce, your favorite hot sauce, chestnuts and Splenda. Mix thoroughly to combine and set aside for later use.

2. Then spray a large sized skillet with a generous amount of cooking spray. Set over medium heat.

3. Once your skillet is hot to the touch, add in your onions and cook until they are fragrant and soft to the touch.

4. Add in your garlic and cook for an additional until fragrant.

5. Increase your heat to medium or high heat. Then add in your chicken, ginger and dash of salt. Stir thoroughly to combine. Cook until your chicken is no longer pink in color.

6. Add in your chestnut mixture and stir again to combine. Cook for at least 2 minutes.

7. Add in your oil and remove from heat.

8. Serve your mixture upon your lettuce leaves. Top off with your onion and cucumber. Serve immediately and enjoy.

Hearty Chicken Cheesesteak Wrap

Here is yet another hearty chicken recipe that you are not going to be able to resist. Best during the summer holidays, you can easily serve this dish up during a family picnic or whenever you are watching fireworks. Either way you are going to love it.

Makes: 1 Serving

Total Prep Time: 25 Minutes

Ingredients:

- ¼ Pound of Chicken Breast, Boneless, Skinless and Trimmed of Fat
- ¼ Cup of Onions, Finely Chopped
- ¼ Cup of Green Peppers, Thinly Sliced
- ¼ Cup of Mushrooms, Thinly Sliced
- 1, ¾ Wedge of Swiss Cheese, Light
- 1 Flour Tortilla, Whole Wheat Variety
- 2 tsp. of Chili Peppers, Hot and Thinly Sliced

Directions:

1. The first thing that you will want to do is thinly slice up your chicken into strips.

2. Place a large sized skillet over medium to high heat. Generously grease it with some cooking spray.

3. Once your skillet is hot enough add in your onion and chicken. Cook until your onions are translucent and your chicken is fully cooked through.

4. Add in your mushrooms and green peppers and continue to cook until they are tender to the touch.

5. Then place your tortilla between 2 paper towels and place into your microwave for the next 20 seconds.

6. After this time lay your tortilla on a plate. Spoon your cheese in a thin strip in the middle.

7. Top off with your peppers, chicken, onions and mushrooms

8. Add your chili peppers and fold over. Serve right away and enjoy.

Healthy Black Bean and Pumpkin Soup

If you are looking for a healthy and smooth soup recipe to enjoy, you can't go wrong with this dish. It is the perfect dish to make during the holiday season or whenever you are feeling a bit under the weather.

Makes: 6 Servings

Total Prep Time: 35 Minutes

Ingredients:

- 2 Tbsp. of Olive Oil, Extra Virgin
- 1 Onion, Medium in Size and Chopped Finely
- 4 Cloves of Garlic, Minced
- 1 Tbsp. of Cumin, Ground
- 1 tsp. of Chili, Powdered Variety
- ½ tsp. of Black Pepper, For Taste
- 2, 15 Ounce Cans of Black Beans, Rinsed and Drained
- 1 Cup of Tomatoes, Canned Variety and Finely Diced
- 2 Cups of Beef Broth
- 1, 16 Ounce Can of Pumpkin Puree

Directions:

1. The first thing that you will want to do is heat up your oil in a large sized soup pot over medium heat. Once the soup pot is hot enough add in your onions, cumin, garlic, powdered chili and dash of pepper. Cook until soft to the touch.

2. Add in your black beans, pumpkin, broth and tomatoes. Stir thoroughly to combine.

3. Reduce the heat to low and simmer for the next 25 minutes or until your soup is thick in consistency.

4. After this time pour your soup into a food processor and blend on the highest setting until smooth in consistency.

5. Pour back into your pot and heat up until piping hot.

6. Remove from heat and serve right away.

Spiced Deviled Eggs

Here is a delicious appetizer recipe that you are going to want to share during your next family gathering. These tasty treats are incredibly delicious and packed full of a spicy flavor that you won't be able to resist.

Makes: 3 Servings

Total Prep Time: 4 Servings

Ingredients:

- 6 Eggs, Hardboiled Variety
- 2 Tbsp. of Horseradish Sauce, Creamy Variety
- ½ tsp. of Dill, Fresh
- ¼ tsp. of Mustard, Spicy Variety
- 1/8 tsp. of Salt, For Taste
- Dash of Salt and Pepper, For Taste

Directions:

1. First peel your eggs and slice them lengthwise.

2. Place three of your egg yolks into your mixing bowl while setting the egg whites aside for later use.

3. Add your horseradish sauce to your egg yolks along with your fresh dill, mustard and dash of salt. Mash your egg yolk mixture thoroughly.

4. Spoon this filling into your egg white halves and season with a dash of pepper and paprika.

Stir Fry Ginger Beef

Here is yet another Asian inspired recipe that I know you won't be able to get enough of. Easy to make and only requires a handful of ingredients, this is a great dish for those who are running short on time.

Makes: 6 Servings

Total Prep Time: 15 Minutes

Ingredients:

- 1 Pound of Flank Steak, Cut into Thin Strips
- 2 tsp. of Ginger, Ground Variety
- 2 Cloves of Garlic, Minced
- 6 Ounces of Beef Broth, Fat Free
- ¼ Cup of Hoisin Sauce
- 3 Tbsp. of Soy Sauce, Your Favorite Kind
- 1 Tbsp. of Cornstarch
- 1 tsp. of Oil, Canola Variety
- ¼ tsp. of Red Pepper Flakes, Crushed
- 3 Ounces of Broccoli Florets, Fresh
- ½ of A Green Pepper, Medium in Size and Cut into Strips
- ½ Cup of Brown Rice, Instant Variety
- 2 Stalks of Bok Choy, Medium in Size and Sliced Thinly
- 1, 8 Ounce Can of Chestnuts, Water Variety and Thinly

Directions:

1. Use a large sized mixing bowl and stir together your ginger, garlic and steak until thoroughly mixed. Set this mixture aside.

2. Next prepare your rice according to the directions on the package.

3. Then combine your broth, favorite soy sauce, cornstarch and hoisin sauce together in a medium sized bowl. Stir thoroughly until dissolved.

4. Use a large sized wok and heat up some oil over medium heat. Once the oil is hot enough add in your pepper flakes. Stir to coat in the oil.

5. Add in your steak and cook for the next 5 minutes or until brown in color. Make sure that you stir your steak constantly. Once brown remove from heat and set aside for later use.

6. Add in your broccoli, bell pepper and carrots into your pan. Cook for the next 2 to 3 minutes or until tender to the touch.

7. Next add in your bok choy and chestnuts. Stir again to incorporate and continue to cook for the next 1 to 2 minutes or until your bok choy is crispy to the touch.

8. Make a well in the center of your mixture and pour in your broth. Continue to cook for the next 2 minutes or until your broth is thick in consistency.

9. Add in your beef and remove from heat. Stir thoroughly to combine and serve while your dish is warm.

Slow Cooker Style Chicken Tikka Masala

Here is yet another unique and exotic dish that you are going to love. While it is a bit heartier, this is still a dish you can enjoy while on your gastric surgery diet that you don't need to feel guilty of.

Makes: 10 Servings

Total Prep Time: 4 to 8 Hours

Ingredients:

- 3 Pounds of Chicken Breast, Boneless and Skinless Variety
- 1 Onion, Large in Size and Finely Diced
- 4 Cloves of Garlic, Minced
- 2 Tbsp. of Ginger, Fresh and Minced
- 1, 29 Ounce Can of Tomato Puree
- 1 ½ Cups of Yogurt, Greek Variety and Plain
- 2 Tbsp. of Olive Oil, Extra Virgin Variety
- 2 Tbsp. of Garam Masala
- 1 Tbsp. of Cumin
- ½ Tbsp. of Paprika
- ¾ tsp. of Cinnamon, Ground
- ¾ tsp. of Black Pepper, For Taste
- 1 to 3 tsp. of Cayenne Pepper
- 2 Bay Leaves, Fresh
- Some Cilantro, For Topping and Roughly Chopped

Directions:

1. First place all of your ingredients except for your cilantro into a large sized mixing bowl. Stir thoroughly to evenly combine.

2. Spoon this mixture carefully into your slow cooker.

3. Cover and cook on the lowest setting for the next 8 hours or on the highest setting for the next 4 hours.

4. After this time remove your bay leaves and serve with your cilantro as a topping. Enjoy.

Classic Baked Tomatoes

If you are looking for a healthy and delicious snack to enjoy, you can't go wrong with this recipe. Feel free to serve these tasty tomatoes during your next family gathering or make it whenever you want to spoil yourself.

Makes: 6 Servings

Total Prep Time: 1 Hour

Ingredients:

- 5 to 6 Tomatoes, Large in Size
- Some Cooking Spray
- ¼ Cup of Parmesan Cheese, Low in Fat
- Some Greek Seasoning, For Taste
- ¼ Cup of Pine Nuts, Optional

Directions:

1. The first thing that you will want to do is preheat your oven to 350 degrees.

2. While your oven is heating up slice your tomatoes in half lengthwise and place onto a generously greased baking sheet.

3. Spray the surface of your tomatoes with some cooking spray.

4. Top off with your cheese, nuts and Greek seasoning.

5. Place into your oven to bake for the next 50 minutes.

6. After this time remove from oven and allow to cool slightly before serving.

Simple Egg Muffin

If you are looking for a light and hearty breakfast recipe to enjoy, then this is the perfect dish for you. This is the perfect dish to make if you if you are running short on time and need to take breakfast on the go with you.

Makes: 12 Servings

Total Prep Time: 35 Minutes

Ingredients:

- 6 Eggs, Large in Size and Beaten
- 12 Slices of Bacon, Turkey Variety and Pre-cooked
- ¾ Cup of Swiss Cheese, Shredded and Low in Fat
- ½ Cup of Milk, 1% Variety
- ¼ tsp. of Salt, For Taste
- ¼ tsp. of Pepper, For Taste
- ¼ tsp. of Italian Seasoning

Directions:

1. The first thing that you will want to do is spray a muffin tin with a generous amount of cooking spray.

2. Then preheat your oven to 350 degrees.

3. Next place 3 slices of bacon into the bottom of each muffin cup.

4. Use a large sized mixing bowl and mix together your remaining ingredients except for your cheese until evenly blended. Spoon at least ¼ cup of this mixture into each muffin cup.

5. Top off with your cheese on each muffin mixture.

6. Place into your oven to bake for the next 20 to 25 minutes or until your eggs are completely set.

7. Remove and allow to cool slightly before serving. Enjoy.

Vegetarian Cheesy Chili

This is the perfect chili recipe to put together if you are feeling under the weather or need to be warmed up on a cold winter's night. For the tastiest results feel free to serve this dish up with some crackers.

Makes: 8 Servings

Total Prep Time: 25 Minutes

Ingredients:

- 2 Cloves of Garlic, Minced
- 2 tsp. of Olive Oil, Extra Virgin Variety
- 1 Green Bell Pepper, Large in Size and Finely Diced
- 1 Cup of Onion, Finely Chopped
- ½ Pound of Mushrooms, Thinly Sliced
- 14.5 Ounce Can of Tomatoes, Finely Diced
- 1, 8 Ounce Can of Tomato Sauce
- 2 Tbsp. of Chili, Powdered Variety
- 1 Zucchini, Medium in Size and Thinly Sliced
- 2, 15 Ounce Cans of Kidney Beans, Red in Color and Rinsed
- 1, 10 Ounce Pack of Corn, Frozen Variety
- 1 Cup of Cheddar Cheese, Low in Fat and Finely Shredded

Directions:

1. First heat up some olive oil in a large sized skillet placed over medium heat. Once the oil is hot enough add in your garlic and cook for at least one minute.

2. Then add in your green peppers, mushrooms and onions and cook until they are all tender to the touch. This should take at least 10 to 15 minutes.

3. After this time add in your tomato sauce, tomatoes and powdered chili. Bring this mixture to a rolling boil.

4. Once your mixture is boiling reduce the heat to low and add in your beans and zucchini. Allow to simmer for the next 10 to 15 minutes.

5. Add in your corn and at least half a cup of your cheese. Stir thoroughly to combine.

6. Continue to simmer for another 10 to 15 minutes before removing from heat.

7. Serve and top off with some more cheddar cheese. Enjoy.

Fruit Packed Breakfast Wrap

Want a filling breakfast that is also incredibly healthy for you? If so, this is one recipe you need to try for yourself. It is surprisingly delicious I know you will want to enjoy it every morning.

Makes: 1 Serving

Total Prep Time: 5 Minutes

Ingredients:

- 1 Tortilla, Whole Wheat Variety
- 3 Tbsp. of Ricotta Cheese, Regular Variety
- 1 Tbsp. of Jelly, Strawberry Flavored and Low in Sugar
- 1/3 Cup of Strawberries, Fresh and Thinly Sliced

Directions:

1. First spread your ricotta cheese and jelly on your tortilla.

2. Sprinkle your strawberries over your cheese and jelly.

3. Roll up your tortilla burrito style and enjoy right away.

Veggie Style Pizza

Love pizza? Then this is the perfect dish for you to make. It is packed full of healthy vegetables and cool ranch, making for a filling and hearty pizza dish you won't be able to resist.

Makes: 8 Servings

Total Prep Time: 10 Minutes

Ingredients:

- 2 Wraps, Low Carb Variety
- ½ Cup of Cream Cheese, Chive and Onion Variety and Reduced in Fat
- ½ Cup of Sour Cream, Light
- 1 Package of Ranch Dressing, Dried
- 1/8 Cup of Carrots, Finely Shredded
- ¾ Cup of Broccoli, Raw
- ¾ Cup of Tomatoes, Finely Diced
- 1/8 Cup of Green Peppers, Finely Diced
- 1/8 Cup of Cucumbers, Finely Diced
- ¾ Cup of Monterey Jack and Colby Cheese, Finely Shredded
- ½ Cup of Black Olives, Thinly Sliced

Directions:

1. The first thing that you will want to do is mix together your cream cheese, sour cream and ranch in a medium sized bowl.

2. Spread this mixture evenly on your tortillas.

3. Top off with your veggie and olives.

4. Sprinkle your cheese over the top

5. Cut your pizza into four equal sized pieces and serve whenever you are ready.

Simple Turkey Turnovers

Here is a simple recipe for you to make, especially if you have a bunch of leftovers. For the tastiest results I highly recommend serving this with a side of cranberry sauce to use as a dipping sauce.

Makes: 24 Servings

Total Prep Time: 15 Minutes

Ingredients:

- 1 Envelope of Onion Soup, Dried
- 1 Pound of Turkey, Ground and Breast Only
- 1 Cup of Cheese, 2% Variety, Finely Shredded and Low in Fat
- 3 Tubes of Crescent Rolls, Reduced in Fat

Directions:

1. The first thing that you will want to do is preheat your oven to 350 degrees.

2. While your oven is heating up mix your dried soup mix with your turkey in a large sized skillet placed over medium heat. Cook until your meat is brown in color.

3. Slowly add in your cheese.

4. Then unroll your dough, separate your rolls and cut into small sized triangles.

5. Place a spoonful of your meat mixture into each triangle.

6. Fold over and seal the edges with your fingertips. Place onto a generously greased cookie sheet.

7. Place into your oven to bake for the next 15 minutes.

Turkey and Bean Enchiladas

If you are craving authentic Spanish cuisine, then this is a great dish for you to make. This dish makes for a great tasting meal to enjoy any day of the week.

Makes: 4 Servings

Total Prep Time: 30 Minutes

Ingredients:

- 6 Scallions, Medium in Size and White and Green Parts Finely Chopped
- 2 Cups of Turkey Meat, Skinless and Boneless Variety and Cut into Small Sized Cubes
- 1, 15 Ounce Can of Pinto Beans, Drained and Rinsed
- 1 Cup of Enchilada Sauce, Your Favorite Kind
- 4 Tortillas, Medium in Size, Low Carb and Fat Free
- ½ Cup of Mexican Style Cheese, Finely Shredded and Reduce in Fat

Directions:

1. First preheat your oven to 350 degrees.

2. While your oven is heating use a medium sized bowl and thoroughly combine your scallions, ground turkey, beans and at least half of a cup of your enchilada sauce.

3. Spoon your turkey filling into each tortilla and roll up burrito style.

4. Place your tortillas with the seam side down into a large sized baking dish.

5. Pour your remaining enchilada sauce over the top and top off with your shredded cheese.

6. Cover with some aluminum foil and bake for the next 20 minutes or until your cheese is bubbly and your enchiladas are piping hot.

7. Remove from your oven and serve whenever you are ready.

Healthy Stuffed Cabbage Rolls

Here is yet another healthy dish that I know you are going to love. Feel free to serve this dish up as your main meal or to enjoy as a tasty snack throughout the day.

Makes: 6 Servings

Total Prep Time: 50 Minutes

Ingredients:

- 1 Head of Cabbage, With Individual Leaves Removed
- 1/3 Cup of Brown Rice, Instant Variety
- 1 tsp. of Olive Oil, Extra Virgin Variety
- ½ of an Onion, Medium in Size and Finely Diced
- 2 Carrots, Medium in Size and Finely Diced
- 1 Pound of Turkey, Lean and Ground
- 2 tsp. of Garlic, Powdered Variety
- 2 tsp. of Italian Seasoning
- 2 Cups of Tomato Sauce

Directions:

1. The first thing that you will want to do is preheat your oven to 350 degrees.

2. While your oven is heating up blanch your cabbage for at least 30 seconds. Remove and set aside for later use.

3. Then cook up your rice according to the directions on the package. Once cooked, set aside for later use.

4. Next use a large sized skillet and heat up your oil over medium heat. Once the oil is hot enough add in your carrots and onions. Cook while stirring frequently to ensure that both are soft to the touch and caramelized.

5. Add in your turkey and continue to cook until your turkey is brown in color.

6. Add in your garlic powder and Italian seasoning. Stir to thoroughly combine.

7. Mix together your turkey mixture with your rice until evenly mixed. Remove from heat.

8. Spoon at least half a cup of your mixture into each leaf of lettuce. Roll up burrito style and place into a large sized baking side with the seam side facing down.

9. Pour your tomato sauce over the top of your cabbage rolls.

10. Place into your oven to bake for the next 35 to 45 minutes.

11. After this time remove from your oven and allow to cool for at least 5 to 10 minutes before serving. Enjoy.

Moist and Succulent Chicken

If you have ever made chicken before for it to only turn out dry, then this is one recipe that you need to try making for yourself. Just as the name implies this dish will make some of the tastiest and most succulent chicken you will ever come across.

Makes: 12 Servings

Total Prep Time: 50 Minutes

Ingredients:

- 3 Pounds of Chicken Breasts, Boneless and Skinless Variety
- 1 ¼ Cups of Bread Crumbs, Italian Variety
- ½ Cup of Mayonnaise, Light Variety

Directions:

1. The first thing that you will want to do is preheat your oven to 425 degrees.

2. While your oven is heating up, brush your mayonnaise directly onto your chicken.

3. Then place your breadcrumbs onto a large sized plate. Roll your chicken in your breadcrumbs until thoroughly coated.

4. Place your coated chicken into a large sized baking dish.

5. Place into your oven to bake for the next 40 to 45 minutes or until your chicken is fully cooked through.

6. After this time remove from your oven and allow to cool slightly before serving.

Conclusion

Well there you have it!

Hopefully by the end of this book you have learned that having weight loss surgery is not necessarily something that you should be afraid of. I also hope that you have learned when it comes to eating after your surgery, you don't have to sacrifice anything in the process. Hopefully you have learned exactly that with the 25 different gastric bypass friendly recipes I have given you in this book.

So, what is the next step for you to take?

Well, the next step for you to take is to take it easy. Remember, after surgery you do not want to push yourself too hard. Take all of the time you need to relax. However, if you are up for it, then it is time to begin making some of the recipes you have found in this book. Don't forget to adhere to your doctor's advice and only to eat the bare minimum so you can make the most out of this weight loss surgery.

Good luck!

Author's Afterthoughts

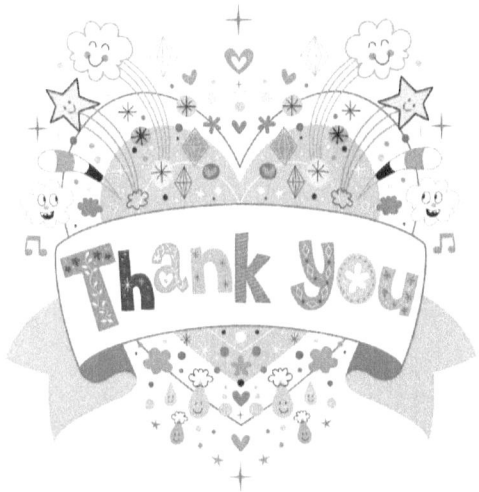

Thanks ever so much to each of my cherished readers for investing the time to read this book!

I know you could have picked from many other books but you chose this one. So a big thanks for downloading this book and reading all the way to the end.

If you enjoyed this book or received value from it, I'd like to ask you for a favor. Please take a few minutes to post an honest and heartfelt review on Amazon.com. Your support does make a difference and helps to benefit other people.

Thanks for your Reviews!

Rachael Rayner